INTERMITTENT FASTING:
101 Guide to Transforming Your Lifestyle Through Diet to Achieve Extreme Weight Loss for Women and Beginners

Minerva Publishing Services & Company

© **Copyright 2019 - All rights reserved.**

The contents of this book may not be reproduced, duplicated or transmitted without direct written permission from the author.
Under no circumstances will any legal responsibility or blame be held against the publisher for any reparation, damages, or monetary loss due to the information herein, either directly or indirectly.

Legal Notice:
This book is copyright protected. This is only for personal use. You cannot amend, distribute, sell, use, quote or paraphrase any part of the content within this book without the consent of the author.

Disclaimer Notice:
Please note the information contained within this document is for educational and entertainment purposes only. Every attempt has been made to provide accurate, up to date and reliable information. No warranties of any kind are expressed or implied. Readers acknowledge that the author is not engaging in the rendering of legal, financial, medical or professional advice. The content of this book has been derived from various sources. Please consult a licensed professional before attempting any techniques outlined in this book.

By reading this document, the reader agrees that under no circumstances are the author responsible for any losses, direct or indirect, which are incurred as a result of the use of information contained within this document, including, but not limited to, —errors, omissions, or inaccuracies.

Table of Contents

PREFACE	**6**
CHAPTER 1.	**8**
WHAT IS INTERMITTENT FASTING?	**8**
CHAPTER 2.	**13**
TYPES OF INTERMITTENT FASTING	**13**
CHAPTER 3.	**19**
THE HEALTH BENEFITS OF INTERMITTENT FASTING	**19**
CHAPTER 4	**27**
MISCONCEPTIONS ABOUT FASTING	**27**
CHAPTER 5	**34**
THE EFFECTS OF INTERMITTENT FASTING	**34**
CHAPTER 6.	**40**
CHEAT DAYS: HOW TO PLAN APPROPRIATELY	**40**

CHAPTER 7.	**44**
EXERCISE AND INTERMITTENT FASTING	**44**
CONCLUSION	**56**
REFERENCES	**58**

Preface

Welcome to "Intermittent Fasting: How to Transform Your Lifestyle Through Diet for Better Health and Extreme Weight Loss." In this book, we will help you to understand the principles behind intermittent fasting and how it can help you.

- If you've tried and failed at every diet fad out there.
- If you're fed up with never having any energy and always feeling tired.
- If you wish there was an easier way to get the body of your dreams without all the calorie counting or drinking endless protein shakes.

Then you are in the right place!

When following an intermittent fasting regime, you simply eat normal amounts of healthy food, but just in a much shorter time frame called the eating window. For example, you eat all of your meals within an 8-hour period each day while eating nothing for the remaining 16 hours.

You may think this sounds hard, but actually, most people find it very simple. Remember that you don't eat while you're sleeping, and this forms a large part of your fasting period.

One of the best reasons to use fasting to lose weight is that it actually helps your body use its fat reserves as fuel, which reduces your body fat.

Fasting shouldn't be looked at as a diet. In reality, it should be used as a permanent adjustment to the way you eat food, combined with eating healthy nutritious foods.

If you are unhappy with your body or your health and are constantly changing your diet without getting the results you are looking for, the intermittent fasting lifestyle may be exactly what you need. The most important part of any successful nutritional plan is having it pertain to your entire lifestyle. This book will not only teach you about the science and benefits of an intermittent lifestyle but will also assist you in reforming other parts of your lifestyle, including exercise, in order to help you achieve revolutionary results.

Fasting is not recommended for children (under 18), women who are pregnant or breastfeeding, people with eating disorders or anyone who has a medical condition unless they get the approval of their doctor or a medical professional.

Chapter 1.

What is Intermittent Fasting?

In recent years Intermittent Fasting has taken the dieting, health and fitness world by storm. The reason for the popularity of intermittent fasting is undoubtedly its simplicity, quick results and numerous health benefits.

Although you may have heard about intermittent fasting, you might still be left wondering what it is and how to do it, so let's take a closer look and find out.

The Principals of Intermittent Fasting

Intermittent fasting is quite simply and eating pattern that revolves on a cycle between times that you are eating and times you are not eating or fasting.

Although intermittent fasting doesn't, in principle, involve any form of food restriction, calorie counting or food group elimination, it is advisable to remember that for best results from intermittent fasting a healthy balanced diet should also be incorporated.

There are various "cycles" of intermittent fasting, which we will look at in more detail in the next chapter, but to give you a basic idea, it is usual for people to fast daily.

We all fast naturally when we sleep at night. During that time our body functions on the energy provided by our food intake the previous day and don't require any further food while we are sleeping. This is why the first meal of the day is called "Break*fast*" as we are breaking our overnight fast.

When you are practicing intermittent fasting, most people choose to extend this fasting period and not eat their first meal until later in the day, perhaps at lunchtime.

You may wonder how you would cope without eating breakfast but, in fact, adapting your body to intermittent fasting is fairly easy to achieve. It is common after the first week of fasting to have increased energy levels and not, as you might imagine, reduced ones.

Many people think that they would suffer from hunger, and although this can be true, to begin with, it soon passes as your body adapts to your new eating cycle.

While you are in a fasting period you cannot eat, but you can drink zero calorie drinks such as water, black coffee and tea, infusions or calorie-free beverages (although these commercial beverages are not recommended as they often contain ingredients that are very bad for your health).

The taking of supplements during your fast is

generally permitted, providing they are calorie free.

Why You Should Fast

In truth, fasting isn't new at all. In fact, we have been doing it for thousands of years. Before modern times, when food has become an easily accessible commodity for most, it was often a great deal harder to come by. During the winter months, food could be very scarce and even eating a single meal a day was often not possible. In these times man feasted in times of plenty, but also often starved in times of hardship.

Some religions also advocate fasting as part of their faith, including Christianity, Buddhism, and Islam.

When we are sick, we instinctively fast, so, as you see, in reality, there is nothing unusual or unnatural about fasting at all.

Fasting changes many of our body's processes. It safeguards us during times of famine so that our bodies can continue to thrive. This is done through changes in our genes and hormone levels and also provokes changes to our cellular repair processes.

When we have undergone fasting, our blood glucose levels and insulin levels are significantly reduced. We also see increases in human growth hormone. This can help us in two ways; it can help us to lose weight, as it automatically reduces our calorie intake, and to use more fat for energy. It also gives us a range of metabolic health benefits.

Evidence suggests that regular intermittent fasting can increase longevity, protect us from diseases such as type II diabetes, cancer, heart disease, Alzheimer's and more besides.

For some people who have struggled with other diets, they find intermittent fasting is the perfect answer, it is straightforward and easy to do and it gives good results quickly. Essentially, it's a perfect "life hack" making weight loss simpler, as well as giving other added health benefits. Not to mention the amount of time saved preparing meals, and money saved buying food.

Intermittent fasting is seen as being generally safe to do, provided it isn't taken to extremes. The food you do eat should be healthy, balanced and nutritious and you should still avoid foods that are not considered good for your health, including:

- Processed foods – items made from white flour (bread, cakes, biscuits, pasta), white rice, processed meats such as ham, salami or bacon
- Foods high in saturated fats should be kept to a minimum. Foods containing trans fats should never form part of the human diet
- Foods high in added sugar

A healthy diet should include:
- Unprocessed foods made from whole grains
- Unprocessed organic meat and fish
- Organic vegetables and fruit
- Foods with monosaturated or

- polyunsaturated fats particularly Omega 3
- Organic free-range eggs
- Pulses, nuts, and seeds
- Nut milks

To Summarize

Intermittent fasting is restricting the times of the day when you eat food. It is natural, easy to do and can save you time and money. It can benefit your overall health and help you to lose weight

Chapter 2.

Types of Intermittent Fasting

As we discovered in chapter one, intermittent fasting involves periods of fasting and periods of eating. There are several ways to do this, and depending on your reason for using intermittent fasting, it is a good idea to choose a way that seems to best suit your lifestyle and personality. By this I mean if you are someone who can be very dedicated to what they are doing one of the tougher regimes may suit, but if you find willpower is a big issue, you may wish to start with a softer approach.

These are some of the more popular intermittent fasting practices:

1. The Diet

This involves fasting for two days and eating normally for the remaining five.

On fasting days, you are only permitted to eat between 500 and 600 calories.

14

This diet first became popular a few years ago and was favored by people who were used to calorie counting.

You are required to decide which two days of the week you will fast in advance and these are not usually sequential. For example, you might decide to fast on a Monday and a Friday.

The problem with this diet is that although you are restricting calories for 2 days you aren't truly fasting, as you can eat the food that gives you the calories at any time of the day. This diet, although relatively easy to do, is not true intermittent fasting and is generally not sustainable.

2. *Eat Stop Eat*

This is where a fast of 24 hours once or twice a weekly is followed. This diet became popular due to its creator, fitness expert Brad Pilon.

In this regime, you are required to fast after eating your dinner and not eat again for another 24 hours. So, if for example you ate your dinner at 7:00 p.m. on a Friday evening and didn't eat again until 7:00 p.m. on Saturday evening then you will have fasted for 24 hours.

This fast cycle can also be done from lunch to lunch or breakfast to breakfast, providing you have a full 24 hours of fasting in between.

Zero calorie beverages are permitted throughout the fast, but no food.

Regular meals should be eaten when you are not fasting.

The main issues with this approach are that to go cold turkey and eat nothing for a full 24 hours can be very difficult. You may also have blood sugar problems that can cause you to feel faint, particularly if you have a job that required physical activity.

Because the fast is only done once or twice a week your body doesn't have time to adapt to the fasting periods, so it is always a shock to the system each time.

It is possible to start with shorter fasts of between 14 or 16 hours and build up to the full 24, but the likelihood is you will be ravenous by the end of your fasting period and this negative association will prevent you from continuing for very long. It may also encourage you to binge eat.

3. Eat Every Other Day Fasting

This fasting regime is exactly as the name describes, eating one day and fasting the next in a continual cycle.

This particular diet has several versions, some which allow up to 500 calories to be consumed on fasting days and somewhere no food can be consumed on fasting days.

The latter method of no food during fasting days is definitely not recommended for beginners, and it still has the disadvantage of your system never fully adapting, because you are either in feast or famine. Due to the harshness of this, it is again difficult to continue for a prolonged period and will cause negative psychological associations.

You can, of course, adapt it to suit you and see what level of calorie intake you find acceptable on fasting days and keep to a healthy diet on non-fasting ones.

4. The Eating Window Method

This is probably the most commonly used and successful of intermittent fasting approaches. Following this eating plan, you are required to fast for a set number of hours per day and are only permitted to eat within a strict eating window.

For example, you may fast from after eating your evening meal that you finished at let's say 7:00 p.m. and not allow yourself to eat again until noon the next day, this is a 17 hour fast with a 7-hour eating window where you can eat lunch at mid-day and your evening meal at 6:30 p.m. in the evening.

Some people prefer to only eat one meal a day, although this can be pretty extreme and beginners would find it difficult to achieve. You can, however, adopt this method to suit you, but you will need a fasting period each day of around 14 hours for women and 16 hours for men (or more), to achieve the best results.

The best part about this method is that most of the fasting is done at night while you are sleeping and denying yourself breakfast is something your body quickly and easily adapts to.

If you want to lose weight rapidly you can also restrict your calorie intake to 1000 a day, or use it in combination with another eating approach such as the Ketogenic diet, which causes the body to use fat as energy instead of glucose.

The eating window method is well tolerated because the body can quickly adjust itself to the routine. It is, therefore, one of the most successful weight loss methods.

If you particularly like eating breakfast then you can change your fasting period and skip dinner instead so you eat your first meal at say 8:00 a.m. and your lunch by 1:00 p.m., giving you an eating window of 5 hours and a fasting period of 19 hours for example.

Drinking water and other zero calorie drinks are fine as it is important to maintain good hydration throughout the day.

A healthy balanced diet should be eaten during the eating window and you should actively avoid "junk" foods.

If you are after an easy to maintain diet, then this could be the best option for you.

5. *The Warrior Diet*

This diet isn't true fasting, as it promotes the eating of small amounts of raw vegetables or fruit before a huge meal at night. It entails spending most of your day fasting (or under eating) and is modeled on a warrior lifestyle, when warriors would be busy hunting, gathering or fighting during the day and would then return home to feast at night.

This was one of the first diets that included a form of fasting and it also relies on the food you consume to be along the lines of the paleo diet, in that it should be raw whole foods that have undergone no processing and still look as they would in nature.

To Summarize

The human body is well adapted to dealing with periods of fasting. In fact, it is probably the most natural form of eating for a human being.

The most successful regime for incorporating fasting into your daily life is one that the body can become accustomed to and just forms part of the natural cycle of eating. This is why the eating window method is the best tolerated along with the warrior diet. It isn't necessary to count calories with either of these options but simply requires that you eat healthy nutritious food.

Lots of people have achieved amazing results using these methods, although intermittent fasting still won't be to everyone's taste. It has been equally successful in both men and women, but may not be suitable for people with eating disorders, due to the risk of under eating and binging.

Chapter 3.

The Health Benefits of Intermittent Fasting

In recent years there much by way of scientific evaluations has been done in intermittent fasting. This has demonstrated that intermittent fasting has a broad range of impressive health benefits. Not only can it help you to lose weight by using fat as energy, but it can also help prevent disease.

1. Weight Loss

The vast majority of people who try intermittent fasting are using it to help them lose weight.

This works in two ways, firstly by reducing the number of overall calories being consumed, and secondly by improving hormone function that promotes weight loss.

This is due to the lowering of insulin levels along with the increase of norepinephrine, which is a growth hormone. This combination increases the metabolic rate and causes body fat to be broken down and used for energy.

The benefit of this double action is that weight loss is being promoted from two sides of the equation. The calories you are using are being increased, and the calories you are consuming are being reduced.

Most individuals see weight loss of between 3% and 8% over a three to twenty-four week period. If you look at it from another perspective and measure your waist circumference to gauge the amount of harmful belly fat lost, it can range between 4% and 7% in the same period.

2. *Reduces Insulin Resistance and Risk of Type 2 Diabetes*

The instance of type 2 diabetes has shown a dramatic rise in recent years. This is thought to be mostly due to poor diet and the consumption of foods that cause insulin levels to become raised over long periods, causing firstly insulin resistance and eventually resulting in type 2 diabetes.

Our body's primary energy source is glucose, which we get from the food we eat. In recent times the amount of glucose-producing foods we consume has increased dramatically.

High carbohydrate processed foods are one of the biggest causes and include breakfast cereals, white bread, white pasta, white rice and products made with refined wheat flour such as cakes, cookies, and pastries. These foods are rapidly broken down into glucose in the body and the sheer volume that floods the system causes a big problem.

Having too much glucose in the bloodstream is bad news, and the body wants to use it up as fast as possible. To achieve this Insulin is released into the body, it helps it use up the glucose for energy and well as taking it to your liver, muscles and (if there is too much, which there usually is) your fat cells.

To give you the basic idea, insulin works by rushing around your body telling all the cells "Hey guys, look, there's lots of glucose here for you to use as energy!" At first, the cells respond and take in the glucose, but quickly they become full and don't want any more, so they start ignoring the message that the insulin is giving them. The body's reaction to this is to release more insulin to try to convince the cells to take the glucose. The insulin levels are raised higher and higher and over a period of time, you become insulin resistant. Eventually, this can lead to type 2 diabetes.

Intermittent fasting can reverse insulin resistance and reduce blood sugar levels, so avoiding type 2 diabetes and kidney damage.

3. Cells, Genes, and Hormones

Fasting causes your body to initiate a cellular repair process and changes hormone levels that allow body fat to be used as energy more easily.

This is what happens during fasting:

Insulin. The level of insulin in the blood drops significantly, allowing fat to be more easily used for energy.

Human Growth Hormone. The amount of human growth hormone circulating in the blood increases to up to 5 times the normal levels. This increase allows fat to be used as an energy source and muscle mass to be *increased*.

Cellular Repair. The cells of the body become more active, repairing themselves and eliminating waste materials.

Gene Expression. Due to the beneficial effects fasting has on gene expression and the function of hormones and cells, it is anticipated that intermittent fasting practices may not only protect against diseases but actually increase longevity.

4. Inflammation and Oxidative Stress

Many chronic diseases, as well as aging, can be promoted by oxidative stress. This is when free radicals, which are unstable molecules, interact with other important molecules such as proteins and even DNA, damaging them.

When combined with a diet that is high in antioxidant-rich foods, intermittent fasting may help your body be more resistant to oxidative stress. Inflammation, which is a fundamental cause of many common diseases, can also be reduced by intermittent fasting.

A study published in the online issue 16 of Nature Medicine, describes how β-hydroxybutyrate inhibits a complex set of proteins known as inflammasome, particularly NLRP3. The inflammasome is responsible for driving inflammatory response in disorders such as type 2 diabetes, Alzheimer's disease, autoimmune diseases, atherosclerosis, and other autoinflammatory disorders.

5. *Heart Health*

The biggest killer in the world is currently heart disease. Intermittent fasting can improve many of the risk factors associated with heart disease, including LDL cholesterol levels, blood pressure, triglycerides, inflammation, and blood sugar levels. Making a useful way to help prevent the disease long term. This is particularly useful for people who have a family history of heart disease.

Unfortunately, because intermittent fasting is of no interest to the pharmaceutical industry (because they can't make money from it), very little study has been done on humans to ascertain the full effects that intermittent fasting can provide. To really understand the full potential a lot more human trials need to be done.

6. *Cellular Repair*

Cellular repair, known as autophagy, is stimulated by fasting. Autophagy is when all the dysfunctional and broken proteins that have accumulated within the cells over time are broken down and eliminated. Autophagy can help protect the body against diseases such as Alzheimer's and cancer.

7. *Cancer*

Another disease that seems to have become more prevalent in recent times is cancer.

Cancer is the uncontrolled growth of cells, as the cells auto-destruct mechanism stops functioning and they continue to grow unhindered.

It is thought that when the body is in a fasting state that cancer cells cannot simply "wait out" the fast in the same way as normal cells do. Because they are permanently stuck in "on" mode, they cannot find the nutrients they need to sustain them during a fast. The healthy cells are unaffected, as they simply hibernate during the fast, which cancer cells cannot do.

Fasting is also useful for cancer prevention, as it reduces insulin resistance that is linked to several cancers. It also causes autophagy, where the cells clean out all the garbage, making them healthier.

As with heart disease, insufficient studies have been conducted to show the full potential of intermittent fasting in humans. We are now reliant on individual health associations to initiate the types of studies that are required to further prove the evidence gained to date.

8. Brain Health

The metabolic boost that intermittent fasting provides isn't only good for the body, it is good for the brain as well.

Oxidative stress, inflammation, blood sugar levels and insulin resistance all have negative effects on brain health. Intermittent fasting has been shown to generate new nerve cells that benefit brain function.

A brain hormone, brain-derived neurotrophic factor (BDNF) is increased with intermittent fasting. Deficiency in this hormone has been linked to depression and other mental health problems.

As intermittent fasting can also help to lower blood pressure to normal levels, it is helpful in the prevention of strokes and heart attack.

9. Alzheimer's Disease

Alzheimer's is the most common neurodegenerative disease and it is incurable. Prevention is, therefore, most definitely the best approach.

Patient's with Alzheimer's can benefit and show significant improvements when following short daily fasts.

Because fasting stimulates cell cleansing it is believed that it can help to prevent the occurrence of disease and maintain brain health.

Other neurological diseases such as Parkinson's and Huntington's may also be prevented or improved with intermittent fasting.

As with most other diseases, more scientific research on humans is required to show the full potential intermittent fasting could have

10. Longevity.

Most of us want to live a long and healthy life, and intermittent fasting could be one of the keys to helping you achieve this.

Fasting has been shown to extend the lifespan of rats in the same way as continuous calorie restriction increases lifespan. It was shown in one study published in the Journal of Nutrition, Volume 31, Issue 3, 1 March 1946, Pages 363–375, that rats fasted every other day lived 83% longer than rats that did not fast.

Although more research is necessary on human subjects, intermittent fasting has shown to be greatly popular amongst the anti-aging crowd.

Due to the positive effects on health, it isn't difficult to understand how intermittent fasting can help with an increased lifespan.

Chapter 4

Misconceptions about Fasting

There are many "old wife's tales" surrounding eating, and we will look at some of them here.

1. Skipping Breakfast

Most of us will have had it drummed in from an early age that "Breakfast is the most important meal of the day" or "If you skip breakfast, you'll get fat" and other such nonsense. Although note here that eating breakfast is important for children and children do not tolerate fasting as well as adults do.

The reasoning behind this is, if you don't eat breakfast you'll become excessively hungry, and are more likely to give in to cravings and binge eating.

What we know is that eating breakfast is not essential in adults, and in controlled trials, there is no difference between people who do or do not eat breakfast regarding weight.

2. Lots of Small Meals Are Better For the Metabolism

It is a popular belief that by eating little and often you will help to increase your metabolic rate, and your body will, therefore, use more calories.

Our bodies do use energy all of the time, and the energy used to digest and absorb nutrients from the food we eat also uses small amounts of energy. The theory here is that by eating regular small meals your body will use up more of the energy provided by these meals to digest them than it would if you just eat three square meals a day.

Although this theory sounds as if it could work, it is not actually based on scientific fact, which stipulates it is the **total amount of calories** you consume each day that matter, regardless of how many meals those calories are eaten in. For example, if you ate three meals each containing 500 calories or 6 meals each containing 250 calories the net result would be the same.

3. Frequent Eating Controls Hunger

Some people are natural grazers and seem to have a need to constantly have something in their mouth. For some, frequent meals reduced hunger cravings, while others say that it actually increase their level of hunger. The reasons for this are probably to do with what is being eating and the individual's metabolism.

At the end of the day, there is no consistent evidence to prove eating more often will reduce hunger or the number of calories an individual consumes.

4. Frequent Small Meals Help You Lose Weight

As we have seen in point 3 above, frequent meals neither boost your metabolism nor reduce hunger. In fact, frequent eating has absolutely zero effect on the energy balance ratio and will therefore also have no effect on weight loss.

5. The Brain Must Have a Continual Glucose Supple

It is true that the brain requires glucose to function as it is the fuel our brain uses. However, eating lots of carbs to provide us with this glucose is completely unnecessary and risks spiking our blood glucose levels and increases our chances of becoming insulin resistant.

The body has no difficulty in producing plenty of glucose from using a process known as gluconeogenesis. Although most of the time this isn't even necessary due to the glucose reserves you have stored in your liver in the form of glycogen.

Even people who have endured long periods of starvation and receive very little by way of carbohydrates can produce ketone bodies from fat. These ketone bodies provide the brain with energy and can reduce the amount of glucose it requires significantly.

We have evolved to do this because we would have been subjected, as many parts of the world still are, too long periods of famine. If we hadn't developed this ability to fuel our brains, we would have become extinct.

Some people suffer from a condition called hypoglycemia, which is low blood sugar. If you are one of these people then you should attempt intermittent fasting with caution and build up your body's tolerances gradually over time.

No matter what your physical condition, it is always highly advisable to discuss any diet plans you have with your doctor before commencing them.

Constant "grazing" is not normal behavior for a human. We aren't cows or sheep. We are much more closely aligned to carnivores and are designed to have periods of fasting.

Links have been made and there may be a correlation between the frequent intake of food and damage to health. It is possible that it could lead to liver stress and an increased instance of fatty liver disease. It may also increase the instance of colorectal cancer.

6. Fasting Forces Your Body Into Starvation Mode

Continued long term starvation or decrease in the number of calories being consumed daily will cause your body to go into a state of thermogenesis (starvation mode). This is to help keep you alive as long as possible by using as little of the available reserves of energy than is absolutely necessary. When you are in thermogenesis your body can reduce the number of calories it uses each day by hundreds and happens with almost every type of restrictive diet.

Short term fasts have been shown to temporarily **increase** your metabolic rate. This is caused by the significant increase of norepinephrine in the blood, which instructs fat cells to break down so they can be used for energy. This is why intermittent fasting works so effectively.

7. The Body Can Only Digest a Small Amount of Protein From Each Meal

Somewhere in the mists of time, it was suggested that the human body is only able to digest 30 grams of protein from every meal. For this reason, eating small high protein meals every two to three hours was necessary to gain maximum muscle mass.

There is no scientific evidence to back this up. It does not appear to matter whether you eat lots of small meals or less frequent larger ones. It is just down to the amount of total protein you consume and not the number of meals you spread it over.

8. Intermittent Fasting Causes Muscle Wasting

It is known that general dieting when you are restricting your calorific intake, can cause the body to use muscle for fuel. However, there is no evidence to show that this is any more prevalent with intermittent fasting.

Many bodybuilders use intermittent fasting precisely to maintain high muscle mass while lowering body fat.

9. Intermittent Fasting Damages Your Health

Although some people believe fasting to be harmful, there is no proof. On the contrary, there seem to be many health benefits gained by intermittent fasting. As we discovered in the previous chapter on the benefits of intermittent fasting, not only can it help us lose body fat and reduce weight, it can also improve our health by protecting us from disease and even extend our longevity.

10. Intermittent Fasting Causes Overeating

It is true that many diets can lead us to overeat or start a binging cycle that can be difficult to break.

After you have fasted, it is natural to eat a little bit more than you would have done if you had not fasted. However, because you will be eating less overall (fewer meals), it is very unlikely that your calorie intake will be any higher.

Overall food intake is reduced, due to the fasting periods and the fasting also boosts the metabolism, reduces insulin levels, raises the norepinephrine levels and increased human growth hormone by up to five times. This effectively causes you to use up your fat reserves, not gain more.

Chapter 5

The Effects of Intermittent Fasting

Intermittent fasting, as we have already discovered, can have many positive effects. In this chapter, we are going to delve a little deeper and look at why this is.

1. *Insulin and Type 2 Diabetes*

Insulin is the true cause of obesity and type 2 diabetes. The question for avoiding these things shouldn't be "How do I reduce my calorie intake?" it should be "How do I reduce my Insulin levels?"

The few drugs that are able to lower insulin, come at a price. They are expensive and they can have some serious side effects. A diet that is low in sugar and refined carbs is helpful to some, but often it isn't enough. The real answer to this problem is, as if you didn't already know, intermittent fasting.

The fasting physiology I am going to outline here was written by Dr. George Cahill. He explains how fasting can help us make a gradual shift from using glucose for energy to using fat instead:

Stage 1.

The body at this point is using exogenous glucose for energy, which simply means glucose that is sourced from outside of the body and comes from the food we eat.

As we start fasting the body runs out of this form of glucose and is forced into the next stage.

Stage 2.

The body is now using glycogen, which is glucose stored in the body. The majority of body tissues are still using glucose for energy, but the muscles, liver and fat cells have started to use fat.

Stage 3.

The muscles, liver and fat cells are now using fat exclusively for their energy needs.

Stage 4.

The glycogen stores have by this point run out. The liver and kidneys now have to use a process called gluconeogenesis to produce glucose that is required by the brain, red blood cells and the inner part of the kidney, called the renal medulla.

Stage 5

The brain has now shifted to using ketone bodies that come from the breaking down of fat. The red blood cells continue to use glucose produced by the liver and kidneys.

The glucose in the blood is no longer from exogenous sources (the food we eat) but is made by the body called endogenous sources.

The fat being used is mostly triglycerides, a triglyceride is made from one glycerol and three fatty acids, hence the name.

As you can see, because the body is using its own fat supplies and not glucose for its primary energy source, the insulin and blood glucose levels remain low, but energy levels remain high. It is a total win for people with diabetes.

2. How Fasting Affects the Body While Exercising

The majority of body tissues have the ability to use fatty acids as fuel and it is only the brain and red blood cells that require glucose, which the body makes by using fat. It is at this point that in reality the entire body is fueled by fat and not by sugar.

The effect of this is that the amount of free fatty acids in the blood plasma skyrockets from being almost undetectable when the body is using glucose for energy.

Beta-hydroxybutyrate and Acetoacetate are the Ketones produced to feed the brain. Their production also shows a sharp increase when fasting.

The triglycerides used as energy are broken down into their component 3 fatty acids and glycerol. The glycerol is sent to the liver and converted to glucose in a process called gluconeogenesis to feed the red blood cells and the renal medulla. **The fatty acids feed the body's energy requirements directly**.

As you can see, fasting doesn't actually starve the body and particularly the muscles of fuel as some people believe. The glucose is simply replaced by fats. The upside to this is that the body can sore a practically unlimited supply of fat, but it can only store a very small amount of glucose. This is why when you are using glucose for fuel, your energy levels can be something of a roller coaster, going from high to low very quickly.

When we are fasting regularly and our body has learned to use fat instead of glucose as its primary energy source, the brain is powered almost entirely on ketones.

Contrary to popular belief, this is completely normal and is the way our body was designed to work. Sometimes people confuse this with ketoacidosis, a condition often experienced by type 1 diabetics, where large numbers of ketones are produced even when blood glucose levels are very high. This is due to the lack of insulin and instead of being used for fuel, the ketones just build up which can be dangerous.

In a four day fast, the fatty acids can increase by 373% while the blood glucose can drop from 4.9 to 3.5. Beta-hydroxybutyrate one of the ketones used to power the brain can increase by up to a massive 2527%!

Over four days, there will be a continual increase in adrenalin. But it is, however, the norepinephrine that increases the most, while epinephrine levels remain quite stable. This adrenaline increases energy levels at all times, even when the body is in its resting state, the effect of this is that the metabolic rate is increased dramatically.

So, what does all of this tell us in a nutshell?

1. Adrenalin levels are increased, particularly when combined with regular exercise. The level of maximum oxygen intake (VO_2) is also slightly increased.

2. You recover from exercise faster and build muscle more quickly due to the increased levels of growth hormone.
3. You use up your fat supplies for fuel with fatty acid oxidation.
4. Insulin levels drop.

The net result, is a leaner, healthier body, with improved muscle definition.

Any adult can do this. It will cost you nothing, you don't have to count calories, buy expensive foods or supplements and you will even save time and money because the amount of food you eat is reduced.

3. Cell Cleansing - Autophagy

Fasting causes cellular cleansing, which is particularly beneficial to the brain. This is called autophagy and is, looking at it directly, where the body eats itself. This may sound alarming, but in reality, it is a good thing.

Autophagy is the body's way of cleansing itself so it can detoxify, repair and regenerate. Autophagy reduces inflammation, optimizes brain function and slows aging. It is also believed that autophagy can help with neuroplasticity and cognitive function, this is beneficial for many neural diseases such as Alzheimer's and Parkinson's.

4. Stress Reduction

Tests have shown that fasting improves not only cognitive function but can also improve resistance to stressful stimuli. The decreased inflammation in the brain increases neurotrophic factors such as growth neurons that improve learning and memory. Because fasting causes challenges for the brain, it adapts itself and builds pathways that cope with stress. This has similar results to regular exercise, both of which increase the brain's protein production to promote growth and strengthen synapses and neuron connections. They both also stimulate nerve cell production in the hippocampus region to increase ketone levels to feed the brain. In turn, this increases the number of mitochondria found in the neurons which helps the neurons to maintain connections, improving learning ability, memory and reducing the stress response.

There are also some indications that the DNA repair of the nerve cells is improved with intermittent fasting, which could produce possible treatments for Dementia or Dystonia.

Interestingly this happens regardless or calorie intake. It is the fasting periods that matter.

Chapter 6.

Cheat Days: How to Plan Appropriately

If you are using intermittent fasting to lose weight then there may be times when your fasting regime is interrupted due to circumstances beyond your control. Don't panic, there are ways you can ensure this doesn't cause too much disruption. In fact, cheat days are a good thing as they can help prevent a slowing of their metabolism from a continual process of more calories being used than are being consumed.

A cheat day is a way of fooling the body into believing that it is getting enough calories, which cause an increase in the metabolic rate.

Dieting can also often cause reduced levels of leptin a thyroid hormone that is necessary for fat burning. Using a cheat day can restore leptin to normal levels.

Cheat days are often highly coveted by dieters because it means a break for sticking with the often-intense regime and also because most of us like to be just a little bit wicked every now and then!

1. Why Cheat Days Work Well With Intermittent Fasting

Because you're naturally consuming fewer calories while fasting, due to the small eating window, it is actually quite hard to overdo the calorie intake even when you do cheat.

A typical meal of 1000 calories allows you to eat a cheat meal without necessarily going over your total daily calorie target, and even if you do, it is unlikely to be by much.

What's good about this, is that it doesn't risk much in the way of weight gain, providing you schedule the cheat meal to co-inside with your eating window.

Here's what you should do:
1. Plan your cheat meal to be within your normal fasting eating window.
2. Do a high-rep workout shortly before or after the meal so your body uses the additional glucose calories you consume.
3. Enjoy the freedom of being able to eat what you want, but don't binge!
4. After you've eaten your cheat meal, return to your normal fasting patterns and foods.Eating lots of carbs – even refined ones is not a big issue for a binge meal. They will spike your insulin levels and this, in turn, will cause glucose to be driven into your muscle tissues. If you've done a big workout just before the muscles will use most of this

by turning it to muscle glycogen and it will cause very little by way of weight increase or fat gain.

1. *Leptin*

As I mentioned at the start of the chapter, it is possible to become deprived of the hormone Leptin when on a strict diet of any kind. By restricting calorie intake, the metabolic rate can slow down and having occasional cheat days can help to prevent this. Cheat days will increase leptin levels to normal concentrations and result in a faster metabolic rate.

Cheat days will depend on the goals you set for yourself. If fat loss is your main aim then planning a cheat day as often as once a week or as infrequently as once every three weeks should maintain the results you require. Cheating, if it is properly planned, can actually be beneficial.

Planning is the key to successful cheating. It can be easy if you have a bad day to just throw in the towel and let your emotions take over. This can, unfortunately, result in your eating every bit of sweet, high calorie, unhealthy food you can lay your hands on. This is one of the reasons why meal planning is really important. Knowing what you are going to eat and when makes it much easier to stay on track.

By planning your cheat day meals in advance, you also have some of your favorite treats to look forward, but can also maintain control. This can help to make weight loss a lot more pleasant.

Be reminded, however, that cheat days are not how you should be eating every day, they are AT MOST to be done one time per week. It can often be best to schedule them to be the same day each week, so there is no risk of "confusion."

Intermittent fasting isn't a diet, it is a way of eating. For optimum results, this should become the way you eat – period.

Remember this, DIETS DO NOT WORK in the long term – I will repeat, DIETS DO NOT WORK. Changing your eating habits FOR LIFE do.

Diets don't work because you will always return to your own bad habits when you finish your diet. You will not only regain the weight you lost but more weight besides. The only way to become healthy and keep weight off permanently is to make a permanent change to the way you eat.

Chapter 7.

Exercise and Intermittent Fasting

It is difficult to know when the best time to exercise is when you are using intermittent fasting. Most advice seems to point to exercising immediately before or after a meal is best, especially for anyone suffering from type 2 diabetes or metabolic syndrome.

Exercising when fasting may be good because the chances are your stored carbohydrates (glycogen) will probably be fairly depleted and exercise will deplete them further and help you start using fat as s fuel source instead.

The biggest problem with exercising when you are in a fasted state is that it increases the risk of your body breaking down muscle for fuel. You are also a lot more likely to run out of energy quicker.

If you repeatedly work out when fasting, it may cause your metabolism to slow down and your performance levels to drop.

So, what can you do to avoid these issues?

The success of any exercise or weight loss program depends on how effective, safe and sustainable it is over time. If you want to reduce your body fat and increase or maintain your fitness level then you need to know how to do it safely.

1. When to Eat
If you are planning to do a moderate to high-intensity workout then you should aim to do it shortly after eating a meal. This will help your body tap the energy it needs to work at optimum levels.

2. Hydration
Drinking water is critically important when fasting as it helps clear your body of toxins and hydrates every cell in your body. It is also needed to maintain body temperature, lubricate your joints and keep you healthy.

3. Electrolytes
Electrolytes are electrically charged salts that carry either a positive or negative charge.
The electrolytes we need most for the body are:
- Sodium (positive) $Na+$
- Potassium (positive) $K+$
- Chloride (negative) $Cl-$
- Calcium (positive) Ca^2+
- Magnesium (positive) Mg^2+
- Bicarbonate (negative) HCO_3-
- Phosphate (negative) PO_4^2-

- Sulfate (negative) SO_4^{2-}

Electrolytes are necessary to maintain the voltage across your cell membranes and to carry electrical impulses between nerves and to contract muscles.

The electrolyte concentrations in your blood are managed by the kidneys. When you do a big workout, you will naturally lose electrolytes, particularly potassium and sodium, in your sweat. It is important to replace these lost electrolytes and this can be done by using something like coconut water, which is low in calories and doesn't contain added sugars, unlike most sports drinks.

4. Dizziness

It isn't uncommon to feel dizzy if you push yourself too hard. Especially if you are exercising after a fasting period and haven't yet eaten. This is caused by low blood sugar or dehydration. Ensure you listen to your body and only push yourself as far as is comfortable.

5. Macros

Macros are the percentages of the food groups you eat split between carbohydrates, fats, and proteins.

- Carbohydrates provide 4 calories per gram
- Fat provides 9 calories per gram
- Protein provides 4 calories per gram

If you are doing strength workouts you will need to eat more unrefined carbohydrates on the day of your workout. If you are doing HIIT (High-intensity Interval Training) then you won't need so many carbs. Remember to avoid refined carbohydrates such as cookies, white bread or white pasta and so on.

If you are working out to body sculpt, you should eat high-quality protein after the workout to aid muscle regeneration. While strength training you should eat around 20 grams of high-quality protein with complex carbohydrates within 30 minutes of finishing your workout.

5. *Exercise for Body Type*

There are three body types, Ectomorph, Mesomorph, and Endomorph. Not only do these body types describe how a person looks, but they also help us understand the best forms of exercise to use and the different metabolic factors that influence weight gain and loss between the types.

By understanding your specific body type, you will be able to successfully plan your diet and training regimen.

The right nutrition and exercise can completely change your appearance, regardless of body type.

6. Ectomorphs

People with this body type are often able to overeat, without gaining extra weight. They have a fast metabolism, which helps them stay resistant to weight gain.

The best type of exercise for an ectomorph is short and intense, with the main focus being on working the large muscle groups.

Ectomorphs have the ability to lose fat easily.

Ectomorph Characteristics:
- Slight bone structure, with a delicate frame
- Flat chested
- Small shouldered
- Lean muscled
- Thin
- Have difficulty gaining weight
- Fast metabolism

It can be difficult for ectomorphs to gain muscle mass. Due to their high metabolism and ability to use calories quickly and efficiently, they are better suited to eating a diet that is quite high in carbohydrates. For best results, these should be eaten just before or just after a workout. These should include plenty of fresh vegetables and fruit, some unprocessed starch whole grains.

High-quality protein and fat sources in the form of unprocessed meat, fish, eggs as well as vegetable sources such as lentils, beans, nuts, and seeds.

In order for an ectomorph to gain muscle mass, they would need to do targeted workouts and may require the help of a high-calorie weight gainer, in the form of shakes, which can help.

Ectomorphs can easily tolerate eating junk food on cheat days, but attention should be paid to getting enough protein.

Strength training incorporating a limited amount of cardio is best. Using routines that involve heavy compound movements with minimal isolation for individual muscle groups (heavy weights, low repetition). Supersets can also be beneficial. Carbing up before and after exercise can prevent too many calories being burned.

7. *Mesomorphs*

Sporting an athletic body, with medium bone structure and strong lean muscle mass, the mesomorph is the best body type of those wanting to do bodybuilding and high muscle sporting activities.

Mesomorphs run testosterone high and are often growth hormone dominant. This predisposition aids in muscle gain while maintaining a low body fat ratio.

It is necessary for mesomorphs to maintain better control of their calorie intake as they can gain excess body fat more easily than ectomorphs.

A combination of weight training and cardio is best for body sculpting for those with a mesomorph body type.

Mesomorph Characteristics:
- Athletic build
- Usually hard bodied
- Strong well-defined muscles

- A rectangular body shape with a small waist and hips with broad shoulders
- Find gaining muscle easy
- Can tend to gain excess fat more easily than ectomorphs

Food

A mixed diet of balanced unrefined carbohydrates and high-quality proteins and fats with a macronutrient split of 40% carbs, 30% protein and 30% fat are good for mesomorphs.

A nutritious diet is essential if gaining body mass without fat is desired. To gain the best strong lean muscle foods such as eggs, poultry, seafood, kefir, Greek yogurt, green vegetables, beans, and whole grains can be beneficial.

Most mesomorphs have a reasonable carbohydrate tolerance, so meals that are carb heavy can be tolerated before and after a workout.

Other beneficial foods include fruits, nuts, and seeds.

Training

Mesomorphs tend to be naturally strong and their bodies respond fast to exercise. Regular resistance training with moderate to heavy weights can help build muscle mass. HIIT and compound body exercises in two to three sets of eight to 12 repetitions with a 30 to 90-second rest between sets are also beneficial.

8. *Endomorphs*

With the highest total body mass and a tendency to carry extra fat, along with the largest bone structure, endomorphs tend to be rather on the heavy side.

Endomorphs have a solid, but soft body that gains fat easily. They tend to be shorter and stockier with thick arms and legs.

They have strong muscles, particularly in the upper legs and are good for lifting very heavy weights for short period (deadlifts), or playing in defensive positions in sports.

Endomorphs then to be insulin dominant and have a low carbohydrate tolerance.

Exercise is an important part of the daily routine for an endomorph, they often suffer from a sluggish metabolism, but if educated to eat the right foods and do the right exercise they can maintain a strong, powerful physique.

Endomorph Characteristics:
- Rounded body shape
- Gains fat easily
- Gains muscle easily although it is often undefined
- Usually short and stocky in build
- Finds fat loss difficult
- Generally slow metabolism

Food

Endomorphs should stay away from carbs and ideally work on a macronutrient intake of 25% carbs, 35% protein, and 40% fat. Using a Ketogenic eating style combined with intermittent fasting gives the best results for this body type and it should learn to fuel itself from fat rather than carbs.

All carbs eaten should be dense unrefined carbs including whole grains, quinoa, millet, oats, sweet potatoes, nuts, and seeds.

Training

To reduce fat gain endomorphs, need to use high cardio exercise as well as high repetition weights (low weight high repetition) to maintain a streamlined physique and burn the most fat. Typically, endomorphs should train four or more times per week aiming to increase muscle mass and metabolic rate.

For best results endomorphs should:
- Train for a minimum of 20-minutes each day
- Work the larger muscle groups such as the legs and back
- Choose exercise that requires continuous rhythmic movement such as running, cycling or power walking, and not ones where there is a lot of starting and stopping, such as HIIT or tennis
- Choose an exercise regime that requires moderate intensity

9. Exercise Types

Whatever type of exercise you choose, ensure that you build it up gradually to avoid overdoing things and putting yourself off, or worse, causing yourself an injury.

Try to choose an exercise that you find enjoyable as it will be much easier to continue long-term. If you find you're not enjoying something, then find something else you do like, don't just stop exercising.

There are different types of exercise:

Low Impact

- **Power walking** – this is no gentle stroll in the park, but a purposeful walk that raises heart rate and even makes you break a sweat
- **Cycling, mountain biking or spinning** – getting in the saddle can help your leg strength and aerobic fitness, working your heart and lungs
- **Gym machines** – Cross-trainer, elliptical machine, ski machine, rowing machine or stepper.
- **Swimming** – there is more to do in the pool than just swim, there are various classes you can try out too, water aerobics, paddle boarding, spinning – yes that really is cycling in the water and more. Check out what's available at your local pool

- **Low impact exercise classes** – talk to the instructor

High Impact
- **Jump rope** – getting out the skipping rope and honing your skills is a great way to boost leg strength and aerobic fitness levels, it also makes you light on your feet
- **Running** – start off with a gentle jog, but as your fitness levels grow, add some sprints, hill work, and steps to really notch it up a level or two
- **CrossFit** – this is a training program designed to work around anyone regardless of fitness level, age or gender. It combines many kinds of exercise with nutrition. Find a group near you
- **P0XX** – this is an intense workout program that you can do at home using the DVDs. You will also require additional equipment such as a pull-up bar, dumbbells, resistance bands, and an exercise mat. The program requires you to work out for 1 to 1.5 hours per day and also includes a nutrition program. You are required to take a fitness test before starting P90X and it isn't suitable for the unfit
- **HIIT** – High-intensity interval training. This type of workout combines short burst of intense activity with short rest periods. The idea is to work to your maximum capacity

- for the active periods so you really push yourself to the limit. The workouts are typically around 30 minutes and are suitable for any fitness level. HIIT workout can use running, swimming, cycling, strength training and exercise movements such as squats and push-ups.

10. Stretch Exercise

Yoga, Pilates, and Tai Chi are all forms of stretching exercise. They improve your suppleness and are useful for fine body sculpting. While the intensity level of these forms of exercise is not generally sufficient for using fat. This type of exercise should form part of your weekly routine, but it is the cardio work that will really help you to lose most fat.

Remember that you should always aim to eat shortly before or just after you exercise. This helps your body to burn calories more efficiently and will give you the best results.

Conclusion

Fasting is easy to do. It is simply a matter of eating to a schedule and can be as simple as cutting out food for a specified number of hours per day (not eating from your final evening meal at 7:00 p.m. until 1:00 p.m. in the afternoon of the following day).

Intermittent fasting can help you to lose weight by causing your body to use fat for fuel instead of glucose.

Intermittent fasting can help to prevent diseases such as diabetes, heart attack, stroke, cancer, Alzheimer's and Parkinson's and could even extend your lifespan.

Insulin resistance can be reversed by intermittent fasting.

There are many misconceptions about fasting, most of these are incorrect or only partially correct. By fasting correctly and using planned cheat days you can be sure that you get the best possible results from fasting.

Fasting is beneficial in other ways too. Not only will it help you to lose weight in the form of fat, but it also speeds up your metabolism, balances blood sugar levels (helping you sustain energy throughout the day) and best of all, it causes autophagy (cell cleansing).

No matter what body type you have intermittent fasting can have positive effects, especially when combined with correct exercise and nutrition.

Intermittent fasting can:
- Help you lose weight
- Assist in rebalancing your hormones
- Decrease insulin levels
- Reverse insulin resistance
- Help prevent diseases such as diabetes, Alzheimer's, heart disease and cancer
- Improve brain function
- Reduce stress response

Intermittent fasting is suitable for adults, regardless of age or fitness level. It is not suitable for children, pregnant or breastfeeding women or people with eating disorders. You should discuss any form of weight loss protocol with your doctor or health professional before starting.

We hope you have enjoyed reading this book and that it has helped you to understand and follow an informed intermittent fasting protocol. We wish you the best of luck in achieving the body of your dreams along with excellent health and longevity.

References

https://www.healthline.com/nutrition/what-is-intermittent-fasting
https://www.healthline.com/nutrition/intermittent-fasting-guide#methods
https://www.healthline.com/nutrition/11-myths-fasting-and-meal-frequency
https://news.yale.edu/2015/02/16/anti-inflammatory-mechanism-dieting-and-fasting-revealed
https://www.nature.com/articles/nm.3804#
https://hope4cancer.com/blog/healing-cancer-on-time-how-intermittent-fasting-may-help/
https://idmprogram.com/fasting-and-lipolysis-part-4/
https://health.howstuffworks.com/wellness/diet-fitness/information/question565.htm
https://www.smartdietandnutrition.com/intermittent-fasting-cheat-day-6-tips-to-success/
http://healthandstyle.com/body-type/exercise-for-endomorphs/
https://www.ncbi.nlm.nih.gov/pubmed/24440038
https://www.ncbi.nlm.nih.gov/pubmed/10837292
https://www.ncbi.nlm.nih.gov/pmc/articles/PMC2622429/
https://www.healthline.com/nutrition/10-health-benefits-of-intermittent-fasting
https://www.healthline.com/health/how-to-exercise-safely-intermittent-fasting

http://thescienceofeating.com/food-combining-how-it-works/workouts-for-all-areas/the-3-body-types-explained/

www.ingramcontent.com/pod-product-compliance
Lightning Source LLC
Chambersburg PA
CBHW070432180526
45158CB00017B/978